MW01490008

TABLE OF CONTENT

1.CLASSIC SPAGHETTI AGLIO E OLIO

Prep Time: 10 mins
Cook Time: 15 mins
Total Time: 25 mins
Servings: 4

Ingredients:

- 400g spaghetti
- 4 cloves garlic, thinly split
- 1/4 cup of extra virgin olive oil
- 1/4 tsp red pepper flakes
- Salt, as needed
- Freshly ground black pepper, as needed
- 1/4 cup of chop-up fresh parsley
- Freshly finely grated Parmesan cheese (non-compulsory)

Instructions:

1. As directed on the package, cook the spaghetti in a big pot of salted water up to it is al dente. Set aside 1 cup of of pasta water after draining.
2. In a Big pan, heat the olive oil over medium heat. Add the garlic slices and cook for approximately two mins, or up to golden brown.
3. Cook for 30 seconds after adding the red pepper flakes.
4. Add the cooked spaghetti, oil, and garlic to the pan. To make a smooth sauce, toss to combine, adding the pasta water you set aside as required.
5. Add the chop-up parsley after seasoning with salt and pepper.
6. If preferred, top with freshly finely grated Parmesan.

Nutrition (per serving):

Cals: 400 kcal, Carbs: 60g

Protein: 9g, Fat: 15g

Fiber: 3g, Sodium: 350mg

2.ONE-POT CHILI MAC

Prep Time: 10 mins
Cook Time: 25 mins

Total Time: 35 mins
Servings: 6

Ingredients:

- 1 lb ground beef or turkey
- 1 onion, chop-up
- 1 bell pepper, chop-up
- 2 cloves garlic, chop-up
- 1 (14.5 oz) can diced tomatoes
- 1 (6 oz) can tomato paste
- 2 cups of beef or vegetable broth
- 1 cup of elbow macaroni
- 1 tbsp chili powder
- 1 tsp cumin
- Salt and pepper as needed
- 1 cup of shredded cheddar cheese
- 1/4 cup of sour cream (non-compulsory)

Instructions:

1. Cook the ground beef in a big saucepan over medium heat up to it's browned. Get rid of extra fat.
2. Add the bell pepper, garlic, and onion to the saucepan and cook for approximately three mins, or up to they are tender.
3. Add the chop-up tomatoes, tomato paste, broth, cumin, chili powder, salt, and pepper and stir. Bring to a boil.
4. Lower the heat to a simmer and add the elbow macaroni. Cook the pasta uncovered for 10 to 12 mins, or up to it is soft and most of the liquid has been absorbed.
5. Add the sour cream, if using, and the shredded cheddar cheese and stir.
6. If preferred, top with more cheese and serve hot.

Nutrition (per serving):

Cals: 500 kcal, Carbs: 50g

Protein: 30g, Fat: 20g

Fiber: 5g, Sodium: 800mg

3.VEGETARIAN LENTIL SOUP

Prep Time: 10 mins
Cook Time: 30 mins
Total Time: 40 mins
Servings: 6

Ingredients:

- 1 cup of dried green or brown lentils, rinsed
- 1 onion, chop-up
- 2 carrots, diced
- 2 celery stalks, diced
- 3 cloves garlic, chop-up
- 1 (14.5 oz) can diced tomatoes
- 4 cups of vegetable broth
- 1 tsp ground cumin
- 1 tsp paprika
- Salt and pepper as needed
- 2 tbsp olive oil
- Fresh parsley, chop-up (for garnish)

Instructions:

1. In a Big saucepan, heat the olive oil over medium heat. Stir in the celery, carrots, and onion. Sauté up to softened, 5 to 7 mins.
2. Stir in the paprika, cumin, and garlic. Cook up to aromatic, another one to two mins.
3. Add the vegetable broth, diced tomatoes, and lentils and stir. Bring to a boil.
4. After lowering the heat, simmer the soup for 25 to 30 mins, or up to the lentils are soft.
5. As needed, add salt and pepper.
6. Garnish with fresh parsley and serve hot.

Nutrition (per serving):

Cals: 200 kcal, Carbs: 35g

Protein: 12g, Fat: 5g

Fiber: 15g

Sodium: 500mg

4.SIMPLE BEAN AND RICE BURRITOS

Prep Time: 10 mins
Cook Time: 15 mins
Total Time: 25 mins
Servings: 4

Ingredients:

- 1 (15 oz) can black beans, drained and rinsed
- 1 cup of cooked white or brown rice
- 4 flour tortillas (10-inch)
- 1/2 cup of shredded cheddar cheese
- 1/4 cup of salsa
- 1/4 cup of sour cream (non-compulsory)
- 1/4 cup of chop-up cilantro (non-compulsory)
- Lime wedges (for serving)

Instructions:

1. Heat the black beans in a mini saucepan over medium heat up to thoroughly hot.
2. Combine the cooked rice, salsa, and chop-up cilantro (if using) in a separate bowl.
3. For a few seconds, reheat the tortillas in a dry pan or the microwave.
4. Lay a tortilla on a level surface to assemble. Place a quarter of the rice Mixture into the tortilla's center using a spoon.
5. Top with a dollop of sour cream (if using), some shredded cheese, and a couple spoonfuls of the warmed beans.
6. Fold the sides of the burrito inward, then roll from the bottom to seal.
7. Lime wedges Must be served alongside.

Nutrition (per serving):

Cals: 400 kcal, Carbs: 60g

Protein: 12g, Fat: 15g

Fiber: 10g, Sodium: 600mg

5.EGG FRIED RICE

Prep Time: 5 mins
Cook Time: 10 mins
Total Time: 15 mins
Servings: 4

Ingredients:

- 2 cups of cooked rice (preferably day-old)
- 2 eggs, beaten
- 1/2 cup of refrigerate peas and carrots, thawed
- 2 tbsp soy sauce
- 1 tbsp sesame oil
- 2 cloves garlic, chop-up
- 1 tbsp vegetable oil
- 2 green onions, chop-up

Instructions:

1. In a Big skillet or wok, heat the vegetable oil over medium heat. Sauté the garlic for 30 seconds after adding it.
2. Cook the carrots and peas for two to three mins, or up to they are tender.
3. Pour the beaten eggs into the pan after pushing the veggies to one side. Cook by scrambling up to done.
4. Break up any clumps in the cooked rice before adding it to the pan. Add the sesame oil and soy sauce and stir.
5. Cook, tossing often, up to the rice is well heated, 3 to 4 mins.
6. Serve right away after adding some chop-up green onions as a garnish.

Nutrition (per serving):

Cals: 300 kcal, Carbs: 40g

Protein: 8g, Fat: 12g

Fiber: 3g, Sodium: 600mg

6. BAKED ZITI WITH TOMATO SAUCE

Prep Time: 20 mins

Cook Time: 30 mins

Total Time: 50 mins

Servings: 6

Ingredients:

- 1 lb ziti pasta
- 2 cups of marinara sauce

- 1 cup of ricotta cheese
- 1 cup of shredded mozzarella cheese
- 1/2 cup of finely grated Parmesan cheese
- 1 tbsp olive oil
- 1 tsp garlic powder
- 1 tsp dried basil
- Salt and pepper as needed

Instructions:

1. Set the oven temperature to 375°F, or 190°C.
2. Follow the directions on the package to prepare the ziti. After draining, set away.
3. The marinara sauce, ricotta, mozzarella, Parmesan, garlic powder, basil, salt, and pepper Must all be combined in a big bowl.
4. Combine the sauce Mixture with the cooked ziti.
5. Pour the spaghetti Mixture into a 9 x 13 baking dish that has been oiled.
6. Bake, covered with foil, for 20 mins. After taking off the foil, bake for ten more mins, or up to brown and bubbling.

Nutrition (per serving):

Cals: 400, Protein: 18g

Carbs: 50g, Fat: 15g

Fiber: 3g, Sodium: 700mg

7. SWEET POTATO AND BLACK BEAN TACOS

Prep Time: 10 mins

Cook Time: 20 mins

Total Time: 30 mins

Servings: 4

Ingredients:

- 2 medium sweet potatoes, peel off and diced
- 1 can (15 oz) black beans, drained and rinsed
- 1 tbsp olive oil
- 1 tsp cumin
- 1 tsp chili powder

- Salt and pepper as needed
- 8 mini corn tortillas
- 1/2 cup of red onion, diced
- 1/4 cup of cilantro, chop-up
- Lime wedges

Instructions:

1. Turn the oven on to 400°F, or 200°C.
2. Add salt, pepper, chili powder, cumin, and olive oil to the sweet potatoes. Place on a baking pan and roast up to soft, about 20 mins.
3. In a mini saucepan over medium heat, cook black beans for 5 mins, stirring periodically.
4. In a dry skillet, reheat tortillas for one to two mins on every side.
5. Fill tortillas with roasted sweet potatoes, black beans, red onion, and cilantro to assemble tacos.
6. Top with slices of lime for squeezing.

Nutrition (per serving):

Cals: 250, Protein: 7g

Carbs: 50g, Fat: 5g

Fiber: 10g

Sodium: 250mg

8. TUNA PASTA SALAD

Prep Time: 15 mins

Cook Time: 10 mins

Total Time: 25 mins

Servings: 4

Ingredients:

- 8 oz pasta (penne or elbow)
- 1 can (5 oz) tuna, drained
- 1/2 cup of mayonnaise
- 2 tbsp Dijon mustard

- 1 tbsp lemon juice
- 1/4 cup of celery, diced
- 1/4 cup of red onion, diced
- Salt and pepper as needed

Instructions:

1. Follow the directions on the pasta packet. After draining, allow to cool.
2. Tuna, mayonnaise, Dijon mustard, lemon juice, celery, and red onion Must all be combined in a big bowl.
3. Add the cooked spaghetti and combine thoroughly.
4. Add salt and pepper for seasoning.
5. Before serving, let it cool in the fridge for at least half an hr.

Nutrition (per serving):

Cals: 350, Protein: 18g

Carbs: 35g, Fat: 15g

Fiber: 2g, Sodium: 600mg

9. VEGGIE STIR-FRY WITH RICE

Prep Time: 15 mins

Cook Time: 10 mins

Total Time: 25 mins

Servings: 4

Ingredients:

- 2 tbsp olive oil
- 1 bell pepper, split
- 1 zucchini, split
- 1 carrot, julienned
- 1 cup of broccoli florets
- 2 tbsp soy sauce
- 1 tbsp sesame oil
- 1 tsp ginger, chop-up
- 2 cups of cooked rice (preferably jasmine or brown)
- Sesame seeds (non-compulsory)

Instructions:

1. In a Big skillet or wok, heat the olive oil over medium-high heat.
2. Add the broccoli, carrot, zucchini, and bell pepper. Stir-fry the veggies for 5 to 7 mins, or up to they are soft.
3. Stir in the ginger, sesame oil, and soy sauce. To coat, stir.
4. Cook for a further two to three mins after adding the cooked rice.
5. If preferred, top with sesame seeds and serve hot.

Nutrition (per serving):

Cals: 280, Protein: 6g

Carbs: 45g, Fat: 8g

Fiber: 6g, Sodium: 800mg

10. CHICKEN AND VEGETABLE SOUP

Prep Time: 15 mins

Cook Time: 30 mins

Total Time: 45 mins

Servings: 6

Ingredients:

- 1 tbsp olive oil
- 1 lb chicken breast, diced
- 1 onion, diced
- 2 carrots, split
- 2 celery stalks, chop-up
- 4 cups of chicken broth
- 1 tsp thyme
- 1 tsp rosemary
- Salt and pepper as needed
- 1 cup of spinach (non-compulsory)

Instructions:

1. In a Big saucepan, heat the olive oil over medium heat. Cook for approximately five mins after adding the diced chicken, or up to browned.
2. Stir in the celery, carrots, and onion. Cook for five more mins.

3. Add the salt, pepper, rosemary, thyme, and chicken broth. Bring to a boil, then simmer for 20 to 25 mins on low heat.
4. If using, add spinach in the final five mins of cooking.
5. Warm up and serve.

Nutrition (per serving):

Cals: 200, Protein: 30g

Carbs: 15g, Fat: 5g

Fiber: 3g, Sodium: 700mg

11.STUFFED BELL PEPPERS WITH GROUND TURKEY

Prep Time: 15 mins
Cook Time: 35 mins
Total Time: 50 mins
Servings: 4

Ingredients:

- 4 Big bell peppers (red, yellow, or green)
- 1 lb ground turkey
- 1 medium onion, chop-up
- 2 cloves garlic, chop-up
- 1 can (14.5 oz) diced tomatoes
- 1 cup of cooked rice (white, brown, or quinoa)
- 1 tsp chili powder
- 1/2 tsp cumin
- Salt and pepper as needed
- 1/2 cup of shredded mozzarella cheese (non-compulsory)
- 1 tbsp olive oil

Instructions:

1. Turn the oven on to 375°F, or 190°C.
2. Take out the bell peppers' seeds and slice off their tops. Put them away.
3. Heat the olive oil in a big skillet over medium heat. Add the ground turkey and heat, breaking it up as it cooks, up to browned.
4. Cook the chop-up onion and garlic for three to four mins, or up to they are tender.

5. Add the cooked rice, cumin, chili powder, chop-up tomatoes (with juices), salt, and pepper. Simmer for 5 to 7 mins after thoroughly combineing.
6. Gently press the turkey Mixture into the bell peppers to ensure the stuffing is packed in.
7. The filled peppers Must be put on a baking dish. Top with mozzarella cheese if you'd like.
8. Bake the peppers for 30 to 35 mins, covered with foil, or up to they are soft.
9. Warm up and serve.

Nutrition (per serving):

Cals: 320 kcal, Protein: 30g

Carbs: 35g, Fat: 12g

Fiber: 5g

Sodium: 500mg

12. BUDGET-FRIENDLY SHEPHERD'S PIE

Prep Time: 20 mins
Cook Time: 45 mins
Total Time: 1 hr 5 mins
Servings: 6

Ingredients:

- 1 lb ground beef or lamb
- 1 medium onion, diced
- 2 carrots, diced
- 1 cup of refrigerate peas
- 3 cloves garlic, chop-up
- 1/4 cup of tomato paste
- 1 cup of beef broth
- 1 tbsp Worcestershire sauce
- 4 Big potatoes, peel off and cubed
- 1/2 cup of milk
- 3 tbsp butter
- Salt and pepper as needed

Instructions:

1. Set the oven's temperature to 400°F, or 200°C.
2. The ground beef Must be cooked over medium heat in a Big pan up to browned. Take out extra fat.
3. To the skillet, add the chop-up garlic, carrots, and onion. Cook up to tender, approximately 5 mins.
4. Add Worcestershire sauce, beef broth, and tomato paste and stir. Simmer up to the Mixture thickens, 10 to 15 mins. Add the refrigerate peas and season with salt and pepper.
5. In the meantime, heat a pot of salted water up to it boils. Add the potatoes and simmer for 15 mins or up to they are cooked. Add salt, pepper, butter, and milk after draining and mashing.
6. Layer the meat Mixture in a baking dish that has been oiled. Over the top, spread the mashed potatoes.
7. Bake up to the top is golden brown, about 20 mins. Warm up and serve.

Nutrition (per serving):

Cals: 350 kcal, Protein: 25g

Carbs: 40g, Fat: 15g

Fiber: 5g, Sodium: 600mg

13. GARLIC BUTTER PASTA

Prep Time: 5 mins
Cook Time: 10 mins
Total Time: 15 mins
Servings: 4

Ingredients:

- 8 oz pasta (spaghetti, penne, or your choice)
- 4 tbsp unsalted butter
- 4 cloves garlic, chop-up
- 1/2 tsp red pepper flakes (non-compulsory)
- 1/4 cup of finely grated Parmesan cheese
- Salt and pepper as needed
- Fresh parsley, chop-up (for garnish)

Instructions:

1. Follow the directions on the pasta package to cook it. Save half a cup of of pasta water after draining and setting aside.
2. Melt the butter in a Big pan over medium heat. Cook for one to two mins, or up to aromatic, after adding the garlic and red pepper flakes, if using.
3. Coat the cooked pasta by tossing it in the skillet. To assist the sauce coat the pasta, if necessary, add the pasta water that was set aside.
4. Add salt and pepper as needed and stir in the Parmesan cheese.
5. Serve hot, garnished with fresh parsley.

Nutrition (per serving):

Cals: 300 kcal, Protein: 8g

Carbs: 30g, Fat: 18g

Fiber: 2g, Sodium: 250mg

14. CHEAP CHICKEN ALFREDO BAKE

Prep Time: 10 mins
Cook Time: 25 mins
Total Time: 35 mins
Servings: 6

Ingredients:

- 2 cups of cooked chicken (shredded or diced)
- 1 lb pasta (penne or rotini)
- 1 jar (16 oz) Alfredo sauce
- 1/2 cup of shredded mozzarella cheese
- 1/2 cup of finely grated Parmesan cheese
- 1/4 cup of bread crumbs
- 1 tbsp olive oil
- Salt and pepper as needed

Instructions:

1. Turn the oven on to 375°F, or 190°C.
2. Follow the directions on the pasta package to cook it. After draining, set away.
3. The cooked pasta, chicken, Alfredo sauce, mozzarella, and Parmesan cheese Must all be combined in a big bowl. Add salt and pepper for seasoning.
4. Place the Mixture in a baking dish that has been oiled, then sprinkle bread crumbs on top.

5. Pour some olive oil on top, then bake for 20 to 25 mins, or up to bubbling and brown.
6. Warm up and serve.

Nutrition (per serving):

Cals: 420 kcal, Protein: 28g

Carbs: 35g, Fat: 20g

Fiber: 2g, Sodium: 650mg

15. SPICY CHICKPEA STEW

Prep Time: 10 mins
Cook Time: 25 mins
Total Time: 35 mins
Servings: 4

Ingredients:

- 2 cans (15 oz every) chickpeas, drained and rinsed
- 1 medium onion, chop-up
- 2 cloves garlic, chop-up
- 1 can (14.5 oz) diced tomatoes
- 1 tsp cumin
- 1/2 tsp smoked paprika
- 1/2 tsp chili powder
- 1/4 tsp cayenne pepper (non-compulsory, for extra spice)
- 2 cups of vegetable broth
- 2 tbsp olive oil
- Salt and pepper as needed
- Fresh cilantro (for garnish)

Instructions:

1. Heat the olive oil in a big saucepan over medium heat. Cook the onion for three to four mins, or up to it becomes tender.
2. Add the cayenne pepper (if using), chili powder, paprika, cumin, and garlic. Stir up to aromatic, about 1 min.
3. Add the diced tomatoes, vegetable broth, and chickpeas and stir. Allow the flavors to combine by bringing to a simmer and cooking for 15 to 20 mins.

4. As needed, add salt and pepper. Garnish the stew with fresh cilantro and serve it hot.

Nutrition (per serving):

Cals: 250 kcal, Protein: 12g

Carbs: 40g, Fat: 8g

Fiber: 10g

Sodium: 600mg

16. BASIC TOMATO BASIL SOUP

Prep time: 10 mins
Cook time: 25 mins
Total time: 35 mins
Servings: 4

Ingredients:

- 2 tbsp olive oil
- 1 mini onion, chop-up
- 2 cloves garlic, chop-up
- 1 can (28 oz) crushed tomatoes
- 1 cup of vegetable broth (or chicken broth)
- 1 tsp sugar (non-compulsory)
- Salt and pepper as needed
- 1/2 tsp dried basil
- 1/4 tsp dried oregano
- Fresh basil leaves for garnish
- 1/2 cup of heavy cream or milk (non-compulsory)

Instructions:

1. In a Big saucepan, heat the olive oil over medium heat.
2. Add the chop-up onion and garlic, and cook for approximately five mins, or up to they are tender.
3. Add the crushed tomatoes, vegetable broth, oregano, sugar, salt, pepper, and dried basil.
4. Bring to a boil and cook, stirring periodically, for 20 mins.
5. Puree the soup in a blender or with an immersion blender up to it's smooth.

6. Add milk or heavy cream, if using, and taste to adjust seasoning.
7. Garnish with fresh basil leaves and serve hot.

Nutrition (per serving):

Cals: 160, Protein: 3g

Fat: 10g, Carbs: 17g

Fiber: 3g, Sugar: 9g

17. EASY VEGETABLE CURRY

Prep time: 10 mins
Cook time: 25 mins
Total time: 35 mins
Servings: 4

Ingredients:

- 1 tbsp olive oil
- 1 onion, chop-up
- 2 cloves garlic, chop-up
- 1 tbsp ginger, finely grated
- 1 tbsp curry powder
- 1 can (14 oz) coconut milk
- 1 can (14.5 oz) diced tomatoes
- 2 cups of combined vegetables (carrots, peas, cauliflower, etc.)
- 1 cup of vegetable broth
- Salt and pepper as needed
- Fresh cilantro for garnish
- Cooked rice for serving

Instructions:

1. In a Big saucepan, heat the olive oil over medium heat.
2. Add the finely grated ginger, garlic, and chop-up onion. For 3–4 mins, sauté.
3. Cook for one more min after adding the curry powder.
4. Add the vegetable broth, diced tomatoes, combined veggies, and coconut milk. Bring to a boil.
5. Reduce the heat and simmer up to the veggies are soft, about 20 to 25 mins.
6. As needed, add salt and pepper.
7. Add fresh cilantro as a garnish and serve over cooked rice.

Nutrition (per serving):

Cals: 220, Protein: 5g, Fat: 14g

Carbs: 22g, Fiber: 6g

Sugar: 7g

18. SLOPPY JOES ON A BUDGET

Prep time: 10 mins
Cook time: 20 mins
Total time: 30 mins
Servings: 4

Ingredients:

- 1 lb ground beef or ground turkey
- 1 mini onion, chop-up
- 1 can (8 oz) tomato sauce
- 1 tbsp ketchup
- 1 tbsp mustard
- 1 tbsp Worcestershire sauce
- 1/2 tsp garlic powder
- 1/2 tsp onion powder
- Salt and pepper as needed
- 4 hamburger buns

Instructions:

1. Break up the ground beef (or turkey) while you cook it over medium heat in a Big pan up to it is browned, about 5 to 7 mins.
2. Cook for a further two to three mins, or up to the onion is tender.
3. Add Worcestershire sauce, tomato sauce, ketchup, mustard, onion powder, and garlic powder and stir.
4. Simmer up to the sauce thickens, stirring regularly, for 10 to 15 mins.
5. As needed, add salt and pepper.
6. Use hamburger buns to serve the Mixture.

Nutrition (per serving):

Cals: 330, Protein: 25g

Fat: 18g, Carbs: 20g

Fiber: 2g, Sugar: 6g

19. MEATBALL AND RICE CASSEROLE

Prep time: 10 mins
Cook time: 30 mins
Total time: 40 mins
Servings: 4

Ingredients:

- 1 lb ground beef or pork
- 1/2 cup of breadcrumbs
- 1 egg
- 1 tbsp dried parsley
- 1/2 tsp garlic powder
- Salt and pepper as needed
- 1 cup of white rice (uncooked)
- 2 cups of beef broth
- 1 can (14.5 oz) diced tomatoes
- 1 cup of shredded cheese (non-compulsory)

Instructions:

1. Turn the oven on to 375°F, or 190°C.
2. Combine the breadcrumbs, egg, parsley, garlic powder, salt, pepper, and ground beef (or pork) in a bowl. Shape into little meatballs.
3. Meatballs Must be put in a baking dish.
4. Put the rice, diced tomatoes, and beef broth in a another bowl. Cover the meatballs with it.
5. Bake the meatballs for 25 to 30 mins, or up to they are cooked through, covered with aluminum foil.
6. Sprinkle the cheese on top of the casserole, if using, and bake for a further five mins, or up to melted.
7. Warm up and serve.

Nutrition (per serving):

Cals: 400, Protein: 30g

Fat: 18g, Carbs: 36g

Fiber: 3g

Sugar: 4g

20. BUDGET CHICKEN FAJITAS

Prep time: 10 mins
Cook time: 15 mins
Total time: 25 mins
Servings: 4

Ingredients:

- 1 lb chicken breast, split thinly
- 1 tbsp olive oil
- 1 onion, split
- 1 bell pepper, split
- 1 tsp chili powder
- 1/2 tsp cumin
- Salt and pepper as needed
- 8 mini flour tortillas
- Non-compulsory toppings: sour cream, guacamole, salsa, cilantro

Instructions:

1. In a Big skillet, heat the olive oil over medium heat.
2. Cook the chicken slices for 5 to 6 mins, or up to they are browned and cooked through.
3. To the skillet, add the bell pepper and onion slices. Cook up to tender, 3–4 mins.
4. Season with salt, pepper, cumin, and chili powder. To coat, give it a good stir.
5. Use a microwave or a dry skillet to reheat tortillas.
6. Serve the veggies and chicken on tortillas, with non-compulsory garnishes.

Nutrition (per serving):

Cals: 320, Protein: 30g

Fat: 14g, Carbs: 22g

Fiber: 3g, Sugar: 4g

21.SWEET AND SOUR CHICKEN

Prep Time: 15 mins
Cook Time: 25 mins

Total Time: 40 mins

Servings: 4

Ingredients:

- 1 lb boneless, skinless chicken breasts, slice into bite-sized pieces
- 1 cup of cornstarch
- 1/2 tsp salt
- 1/4 tsp black pepper
- 1/2 cup of vegetable oil (for frying)
- 1/2 cup of red bell pepper, chop-up
- 1/2 cup of green bell pepper, chop-up
- 1/2 cup of onion, chop-up
- 1/2 cup of pineapple chunks (with juice)
- 1/2 cup of white sugar
- 1/4 cup of white vinegar
- 1/4 cup of ketchup
- 2 tbsp soy sauce
- 1 tsp garlic powder
- 1/2 tsp ginger powder

Instructions:

1. Combine the chicken pieces, cornstarch, salt, and pepper in a bowl.
2. In a pan, heat the vegetable oil over medium-high heat. In batches, add the chicken pieces and sauté up to cooked through and golden brown. Take out of the pan and place aside.
3. Sauté the pineapple, bell peppers, and onions in the same pan for two to three mins.
4. Combine the sugar, vinegar, ketchup, soy sauce, ginger powder, and garlic powder in a separate bowl. Cover the vegetables with this sauce Mixture and cook for two to three mins.
5. Stir the cooked chicken to coat it in the sauce before adding it back to the pan. Simmer for a further five mins.
6. Over steaming rice, serve hot.

Nutrition (per serving):

Cals: 320, Protein: 28g

Fat: 18g, Carbs: 17g

Fiber: 1g

Sugar: 15g

22.SPAGHETTI WITH GARLIC AND OLIVE OIL

Prep Time: 5 mins
Cook Time: 10 mins
Total Time: 15 mins
Servings: 2

Ingredients:

- 8 oz spaghetti
- 1/4 cup of olive oil
- 4 cloves garlic, thinly split
- 1/4 tsp red pepper flakes (non-compulsory)
- Salt, as needed
- Freshly ground black pepper, as needed
- Fresh parsley, chop-up (for garnish)
- Finely grated Parmesan cheese (non-compulsory)

Instructions:

1. Follow the directions on the package to cook the pasta. Save a mini amount of pasta water after draining and setting aside.
2. Heat the olive oil in a big skillet over medium heat. Cook the garlic slices for two to three mins, or up to they are aromatic and golden brown.
3. Toss in the drained pasta after adding the red pepper flakes, if using. Coat the spaghetti with the oil and garlic by stirring it.
4. To get the right consistency if the pasta is dry, add a mini amount of pasta water.
5. Add salt and pepper for seasoning. If preferred, garnish with finely grated Parmesan and chop-up parsley.
6. Serve right away.

Nutrition (per serving):

Cals: 450, Protein: 10g

Fat: 20g, Carbs: 60g

Fiber: 3g, Sugar: 2g

23.ROASTED VEGETABLE AND QUINOA SALAD

Prep Time: 15 mins
Cook Time: 25 mins
Total Time: 40 mins
Servings: 4

Ingredients:

- 1 cup of quinoa, rinsed
- 2 cups of water or vegetable broth
- 1 zucchini, split
- 1 bell pepper, chop-up
- 1 red onion, chop-up
- 1 cup of cherry tomatoes, halved
- 2 tbsp olive oil
- Salt and pepper, as needed
- 2 tbsp balsamic vinegar
- 1 tbsp honey
- 1 tbsp fresh parsley, chop-up

Instructions:

1. Set the oven's temperature to 400°F, or 200°C.
2. Combine olive oil, salt, and pepper with the zucchini, bell pepper, onion, and tomatoes on a baking sheet. Vegetables Must be soft and beginning to caramelize after 20 to 25 mins of roasting in the oven.
3. Cook the quinoa in a medium saucepan with water or vegetable broth that has been brought to a boil. Add the quinoa and simmer for 15 mins, or up to the water has been absorbed, while the veggies roast. Use a fork to fluff.
4. To prepare the dressing, combine together the honey and balsamic vinegar in a mini bowl.
5. When the veggies are finished, put them in a big dish with the prepared quinoa.
6. Over the salad, drizzle the dressing and toss to combine.
7. Serve heated or room temperature, garnished with fresh parsley.

Nutrition (per serving):

Cals: 250, Protein: 8g

Fat: 10g, Carbs: 35g

Fiber: 6g, Sugar: 10g

24.EASY BAKED CHICKEN DRUMSTICKS

Prep Time: 10 mins
Cook Time: 40 mins
Total Time: 50 mins
Servings: 4

Ingredients:

- 8 chicken drumsticks
- 2 tbsp olive oil
- 1 tsp garlic powder
- 1 tsp paprika
- 1/2 tsp salt
- 1/2 tsp black pepper
- 1/2 tsp dried thyme
- 1/2 tsp onion powder

Instructions:

1. Set the oven's temperature to 400°F, or 200°C.
2. Using paper towels, pat the chicken drumsticks dry.
3. Combine the olive oil, onion powder, paprika, garlic powder, salt, pepper, and thyme in a mini bowl. Apply this Mixture on the drumsticks of chicken.
4. Arrange the drumsticks on a rack or a baking sheet covered with parchment paper.
5. The drumsticks Must be baked for 35 to 40 mins, rotating them halfway through, or up to the internal temperature reveryes 165°F (74°C).
6. Serve hot, along by your preferred sides.

Nutrition (per serving):

Cals: 240, Protein: 20g

Fat: 15g, Carbs: 2g

Fiber: 1g, Sugar: 0g

25.LOADED POTATO SOUP

Prep Time: 10 mins
Cook Time: 30 mins

Total Time: 40 mins
Servings: 6

Ingredients:

- 4 Big russet potatoes, peel off and diced
- 1 tbsp olive oil
- 1 onion, diced
- 3 cloves garlic, chop-up
- 4 cups of chicken broth
- 1 cup of whole milk
- 1 cup of heavy cream
- 1 tsp salt
- 1/2 tsp black pepper
- 1/2 tsp smoked paprika
- 1 cup of shredded cheddar cheese
- 1/2 cup of cooked bacon bits
- 1/4 cup of green onions, chop-up

Instructions:

1. Heat the olive oil in a big saucepan over medium heat. Sauté the garlic and onions for around three mins, or up to they are tender.
2. To the saucepan, add the chicken stock and cubed potatoes. After bringing to a boil, lower the heat and simmer the potatoes for 20 to 25 mins, or up to they are soft.
3. Blend the potatoes for a smoother soup or mash them a little with a potato masher for a chunky texture.
4. Add the heavy cream, milk, paprika, salt, and pepper and stir. Cook for a further five to ten mins after bringing to a simmer.
5. Add the shredded cheese and stir up to it melts.
6. Garnish with green onions and bacon pieces and serve.

Nutrition (per serving):

Cals: 400, Protein: 9g

Fat: 28g, Carbs: 36g

Fiber: 4g, Sugar: 6g

Prep time: 10 mins
Cook time: 1 hr
Total time: 1 hr 10 mins
Servings: 4

Ingredients:

- 4 Big russet potatoes
- 1 tbsp olive oil
- Salt and pepper, as needed
- 2 cups of broccoli florets (steamed)
- 1 ½ cups of shredded sharp cheddar cheese
- ½ cup of sour cream
- ¼ cup of milk
- 2 tbsp butter
- 1 tsp garlic powder
- ½ tsp onion powder

Instructions:

1. Set the oven's temperature to 400°F, or 200°C.
2. Scrub and wash the potatoes. After using a fork to make a few holes in every, massage them with olive oil and add salt and pepper as needed. On a baking sheet, arrange them.
3. Bake up to soft, 45 to 60 mins.
4. Steam the broccoli florets for 5 to 7 mins, or up to they are soft, while the potatoes bake.
5. Combine the steamed broccoli, sour cream, milk, butter, shredded cheddar cheese, onion powder, and garlic powder in a bowl.
6. After the potatoes are done, slice them open lengthwise and use a fork to gently fluff the insides.
7. Place the broccoli and cheese Mixture inside every potato.
8. Put it back in the oven and bake it for a further five to ten mins, or up to the cheese is bubbling and melted.
9. Warm up and serve.

Nutrition (per serving):

Cals: 395, Protein: 15g

Fat: 19g, Carbs: 47g

Fiber: 5g

27.CHICKEN AND RICE SKILLET

Prep time: 10 mins
Cook time: 30 mins
Total time: 40 mins
Servings: 4

Ingredients:

- 1 lb chicken breast, slice into cubes
- 1 tbsp olive oil
- 1 onion, diced
- 2 cloves garlic, chop-up
- 1 cup of long-grain white rice
- 2 cups of chicken broth
- 1 cup of refrigerate peas
- ½ tsp paprika
- Salt and pepper as needed
- 2 tbsp fresh parsley, chop-up

Instructions:

1. In a Big skillet, heat the olive oil over medium heat.
2. Cook the chicken cubes for 7 to 8 mins, or up to they are browned and cooked through. Take out and place aside from the skillet.
3. Add the diced onion to the same skillet and sauté for 3–4 mins, or up to it is tender. Cook for a further min after adding the garlic.
4. In the skillet, combine the rice, peas, chicken broth, paprika, salt, and pepper. Combine to blend.
5. Bring to a simmer, cover, and cook up to the rice is soft and the liquid has been absorbed, about 18 to 20 mins.
6. After adding the cooked chicken, simmer for a further two mins, or up to well warm.
7. Serve after adding some fresh parsley as a garnish.

Nutrition (per serving):

Cals: 450, Protein: 33g

Fat: 12g, Carbs: 49g

Fiber: 3g

28. TUNA CASSEROLE WITH PEAS

Prep time: 15 mins
Cook time: 25 mins
Total time: 40 mins
Servings: 6

Ingredients:

- 2 cans (5 oz every) tuna in water, drained
- 1 ½ cups of elbow macaroni, cooked
- 1 cup of refrigerate peas
- 1 cup of sour cream
- 1 cup of shredded cheddar cheese
- 1 can (10.5 oz) cream of mushroom soup
- 1 mini onion, chop-up
- 1 tsp garlic powder
- Salt and pepper, as needed
- 1 tbsp breadcrumbs (non-compulsory)

Instructions:

1. Turn the oven on to 375°F, or 190°C.
2. Tuna, cooked macaroni, peas, sour cream, cheddar cheese, mushroom soup, chop-up onion, garlic powder, salt, and pepper Must all be combined in a Big combineing dish. Stir up to the Mixture is uniform.
3. Pour the Mixture into a 9 x 13-inch baking dish that has been oiled.
4. If using, sprinkle breadcrumbs over top.
5. Bake for 25 mins in a preheated oven, or up to the top is brown and bubbling.
6. Warm up and serve.

Nutrition (per serving):

Cals: 410, Protein: 27g

Fat: 18g, Carbs: 38g

Fiber: 3g

Prep time: 10 mins
Cook time: 20 mins
Total time: 30 mins
Servings: 4

Ingredients:

- 1 tbsp olive oil
- 1 mini onion, diced
- 2 cloves garlic, chop-up
- 1 can (15 oz) diced tomatoes
- 4 cups of vegetable broth
- 1 package (9 oz) cheese tortellini
- 1 cup of heavy cream
- Salt and pepper, as needed
- Fresh basil, for garnish

Instructions:

1. In a Big saucepan, heat the olive oil over medium heat.
2. Cook for 4 mins or up to the onion is tender. Cook for a further min after adding the garlic.
3. Add the veggie broth and diced tomatoes and stir. Once it reveryes a boil, lower the heat to a simmer and cook for ten mins.
4. Cook the tortellini as directed on the box, which is typically 5 to 7 mins.
5. Stir the heavy cream into the cooked tortellini. Add salt and pepper for seasoning.
6. Top with fresh basil and serve.

Nutrition (per serving):

Cals: 460, Protein: 18g

Fat: 25g, Carbs: 45g

Fiber: 3g

30.SAVORY BREAKFAST BURRITOS

Prep time: 10 mins
Cook time: 10 mins

Total time: 20 mins
Servings: 4

Ingredients:

- 4 Big flour tortillas
- 4 Big eggs
- 1 tbsp butter
- ½ cup of shredded cheddar cheese
- ½ cup of cooked sausage or bacon (non-compulsory)
- ¼ cup of diced onion
- ¼ cup of diced bell pepper
- ¼ cup of salsa
- Salt and pepper, as needed

Instructions:

1. Melt the butter in a pan over medium heat. Saute the bell pepper and chop-up onion for approximately five mins, or up to they are tender.
2. Scramble the eggs in the skillet up to they are cooked through. Add salt and pepper for seasoning.
3. Spread the scrambled eggs, cheese, salsa, and sausage (if using) evenly in the middle of every tortilla when it has been laid flat.
4. Fold in the edges of the tortillas as you roll them into burritos.
5. Warm up and serve.

Nutrition (per serving):

Cals: 320, Protein: 18g, Fat: 22g

Carbs: 23g, Fiber: 2g

31.VEGGIE-PACKED PITA POCKETS

Prep Time: 15 mins
Cook Time: 10 mins
Total Time: 25 mins
Servings: 4

Ingredients:

- 4 whole wheat pita pockets
- 1 cup of hummus

- 1 cucumber, thinly split
- 1 bell pepper, split
- 1/2 red onion, thinly split
- 1 cup of cherry tomatoes, halved
- 1 cup of shredded carrots
- 1/2 cup of feta cheese, crumbled
- 1/4 cup of fresh parsley, chop-up
- 1 tbsp olive oil
- Salt and pepper as needed

Instructions:

1. For one to two mins, reheat the pita pockets in a pan or toaster.
2. Fill every pita with a Big quantity of hummus.
3. Add the bell pepper, red onion, cucumber, tomatoes, and shredded carrots in layers.
4. Add chop-up parsley and feta cheese on top.
5. Season with salt and pepper and drizzle with olive oil.
6. Serve right away and savor!

Nutrition (per serving):

Cals: 280 kcal, Protein: 9g

Carbs: 38g, Fat: 12g

Fiber: 7g

32. GROUND BEEF AND POTATO SKILLET

Prep Time: 10 mins
Cook Time: 25 mins
Total Time: 35 mins
Servings: 4

Ingredients:

- 1 lb ground beef
- 4 medium potatoes, diced
- 1 medium onion, chop-up
- 2 cloves garlic, chop-up
- 1 cup of beef broth
- 1 tbsp olive oil

- 1 tsp paprika
- 1/2 tsp cumin
- Salt and pepper as needed
- Fresh parsley for garnish

Instructions:

1. In a Big skillet, heat the olive oil over medium heat.
2. Cook up to browned after adding the ground meat. Take out extra fat.
3. Add the garlic, onion, and cubed potatoes to the skillet. Cook, stirring periodically, for 5 to 7 mins.
4. Add cumin, paprika, salt, pepper, and beef broth. Combine to blend.
5. Cook, covered, up to potatoes are soft, 15 to 20 mins.
6. Serve after adding some fresh parsley as a garnish.

Nutrition (per serving):

Cals: 380 kcal, Protein: 27g

Carbs: 40g, Fat: 15g

Fiber: 5g

33. GARLIC PARMESAN ROASTED CAULIFLOWER

Prep Time: 10 mins
Cook Time: 25 mins
Total Time: 35 mins
Servings: 4

Ingredients:

- 1 medium cauliflower, slice into florets
- 3 tbsp olive oil
- 4 cloves garlic, chop-up
- 1/4 cup of finely grated Parmesan cheese
- 1/2 tsp red pepper flakes (non-compulsory)
- Salt and pepper as needed
- Fresh parsley for garnish

Instructions:

1. Set the oven temperature to 425°F (220°C).

2. Combine the cauliflower florets, red pepper flakes, garlic, olive oil, salt, and pepper in a bowl.
3. Arrange the cauliflower on a baking pan in a single layer.
4. Roast up to brown and crispy, turning halfway through, for 25 mins.
5. In the final five mins of roasting, sprinkle the cauliflower with Parmesan cheese.
6. Before serving, garnish with fresh parsley.

Nutrition (per serving):

Cals: 180 kcal, Protein: 6g

Carbs: 12g, Fat: 14g

Fiber: 5g

34. ONE-POT CHICKEN AND SPINACH PASTA

Prep Time: 10 mins
Cook Time: 20 mins
Total Time: 30 mins
Servings: 4

Ingredients:

- 2 tbsp olive oil
- 2 chicken breasts, diced
- 2 cloves garlic, chop-up
- 1 cup of cherry tomatoes, halved
- 2 cups of spinach, fresh
- 8 oz pasta (penne or rotini)
- 3 cups of chicken broth
- 1/2 cup of heavy cream
- 1/4 cup of finely grated Parmesan cheese
- Salt and pepper as needed

Instructions:

1. In a Big saucepan, heat the olive oil over medium heat.
2. Add the diced chicken and simmer for 6 to 7 mins, or up to browned.
3. Cook for a further min after adding the garlic.
4. Add the pasta, salt, pepper, and chicken broth. Bring to a boil.
5. Reduce the heat to a simmer and cook pasta for approximately ten mins, as directed on the box.

6. Add heavy cream, spinach, and cherry tomatoes and stir.
7. Cook up to the spinach wilts, about 2 more mins.
8. Serve after adding the Parmesan cheese.

Nutrition (per serving):

Cals: 420 kcal, Protein: 34g

Carbs: 45g, Fat: 12g

Fiber: 3g

35. VEGGIE CHILI WITH CORNBREAD

Prep Time: 15 mins
Cook Time: 40 mins
Total Time: 55 mins
Servings: 6

Ingredients:

For the chili:

- 1 tbsp olive oil
- 1 onion, chop-up
- 2 cloves garlic, chop-up
- 1 bell pepper, chop-up
- 1 zucchini, chop-up
- 1 can (14 oz) diced tomatoes
- 1 can (15 oz) kidney beans, drained and rinsed
- 1 can (15 oz) black beans, drained and rinsed
- 1 can (15 oz) corn, drained
- 2 tbsp chili powder
- 1 tsp cumin
- 1/2 tsp paprika
- Salt and pepper as needed

For the cornbread:

- 1 box cornbread combine
- 1/2 cup of milk
- 1 egg
- 2 tbsp melted butter

Instructions:

1. In a Big saucepan, heat the olive oil over medium heat.
2. Cook the garlic and onion for three to four mins, or up to they are tender.
3. Cook for five mins after adding the zucchini and bell pepper.
4. Add corn, beans, tomatoes, paprika, cumin, chili powder, salt, and pepper. Bring to a simmer.
5. Cook, stirring periodically, for 25 mins.
6. Make the cornbread combine as directed on the package while the chili cooks.
7. After putting the batter onto a pan that has been oiled, bake it for 20 mins, or up to golden brown, at 375°F (190°C).
8. Serve a piece of cornbread beside the chili.

Nutrition (per serving, chili only):

Cals: 250 kcal, Protein: 10g

Carbs: 45g, Fat: 5g

Fiber: 10g

36.EASY CHICKEN PARMESAN

Prep Time: 15 mins
Cook Time: 25 mins
Total Time: 40 mins
Servings: 4

Ingredients:

- 4 boneless, skinless chicken breasts
- 1 cup of all-purpose flour
- 2 Big eggs, beaten
- 1 ½ cups of breadcrumbs
- 1 ½ cups of marinara sauce
- 1 ½ cups of shredded mozzarella cheese
- ¼ cup of finely grated Parmesan cheese
- 2 tbsp olive oil
- Salt and pepper, as needed
- Fresh basil, for garnish (non-compulsory)

Instructions:

1. Set the oven temperature to 375°F, or 190°C.
2. Use salt and pepper to season the chicken breasts. Coat every breast with breadcrumbs after dredging it in flour and dipping it in beaten eggs.
3. Heat the olive oil in a big skillet over medium heat. Cook up to golden brown, 3 to 4 mins per side.
4. After taking the chicken out of the skillet, put it on a baking sheet. Place mozzarella, Parmesan cheese, and marinara sauce on top of every slice.
5. Bake for 15 mins, or up to the chicken is cooked through and the cheese is bubbling.
6. If preferred, garnish with fresh basil before serving.

Nutrition (per serving):

Cals: 450 kcal, Protein: 50g

Carbs: 25g, Fat: 20g

Fiber: 3g

37. BUDGET BEEF STROGANOFF

Prep Time: 10 mins
Cook Time: 20 mins
Total Time: 30 mins
Servings: 4

Ingredients:

- 1 lb ground beef
- 1 medium onion, diced
- 2 cloves garlic, chop-up
- 1 tbsp all-purpose flour
- 2 cups of beef broth
- 1 cup of sour cream
- 1 tsp Dijon mustard
- 8 oz egg noodles, cooked
- Salt and pepper, as needed
- 2 tbsp olive oil

Instructions:

1. In a Big skillet, heat the olive oil over medium heat. Cook the garlic, onion, and ground beef up to the onion is tender and the meat has browned.

2. Stir thoroughly after adding the flour to the meat Mixture. Cook for one to two mins.
3. Add the beef broth gradually while continuing to stir up to the sauce thickens, which Must take five to seven mins.
4. Add Dijon mustard and sour cream and stir. Add salt and pepper for seasoning.
5. Enjoy the beef stroganoff served over cooked egg noodles.

Nutrition (per serving):

Cals: 500 kcal, Protein: 30g

Carbs: 45g, Fat: 25g

Fiber: 2g

38. EGGPLANT PARMESAN

Prep Time: 20 mins
Cook Time: 40 mins
Total Time: 1 hr
Servings: 4

Ingredients:

- 2 medium eggplants, split into ½-inch rounds
- 1 cup of all-purpose flour
- 2 Big eggs, beaten
- 1 ½ cups of breadcrumbs
- 1 ½ cups of marinara sauce
- 1 ½ cups of shredded mozzarella cheese
- ½ cup of finely grated Parmesan cheese
- 2 tbsp olive oil
- Fresh basil, for garnish (non-compulsory)
- Salt and pepper, as needed

Instructions:

1. Turn the oven on to 375°F, or 190°C. Put parchment paper on a baking pan.
2. To take out extra moisture, sprinkle the eggplant slices with salt and let them for ten mins. Use paper towels to pat dry.
3. Coat every eggplant slice with breadcrumbs after dipping it in eggs and flour.
4. Heat the olive oil in a big skillet over medium heat. Slices of eggplant Must be fried for two to three mins on every side up to golden brown.

5. Arrange the pieces of fried eggplant on the baking sheet. Add mozzarella, Parmesan cheese, and marinara sauce on top.
6. The cheese Must be melted and bubbling after 20 mins of baking.
7. Before serving, garnish with fresh basil.

Nutrition (per serving):

Cals: 350 kcal, Protein: 18g

Carbs: 40g, Fat: 18g

Fiber: 7g

39. ROASTED SWEET POTATO AND CHICKPEA BOWLS

Prep Time: 10 mins
Cook Time: 30 mins
Total Time: 40 mins
Servings: 4

Ingredients:

- 2 Big sweet potatoes, peel off and cubed
- 1 can (15 oz) chickpeas, drained and rinsed
- 2 tbsp olive oil
- 1 tsp paprika
- 1 tsp cumin
- Salt and pepper, as needed
- 1 avocado, split
- 1 cup of cooked quinoa
- Fresh cilantro, for garnish (non-compulsory)

Instructions:

1. Set the oven temperature to 400°F, or 200°C.
2. Add the olive oil, cumin, paprika, salt, and pepper to the sweet potatoes and chickpeas. Arrange in a single layer on a baking sheet.
3. The sweet potatoes Must be soft and golden after 25 to 30 mins of roasting, with tossing in between.
4. Arrange the chickpeas, avocado slices, quinoa, and roasted sweet potatoes in bowls for serving. If desired, garnish with fresh cilantro.

Nutrition (per serving):

Cals: 400 kcal, Protein: 10g

Carbs: 55g, Fat: 18g

Fiber: 12g

40. CHICKEN CAESAR SALAD WRAPS

Prep Time: 10 mins
Cook Time: 10 mins
Total Time: 20 mins
Servings: 4

Ingredients:

- 2 Big chicken breasts, grilled and split
- 4 Big whole-wheat tortillas
- 2 cups of Romaine lettuce, chop-up
- ½ cup of Caesar dressing
- ½ cup of finely grated Parmesan cheese
- 1 cup of croutons (non-compulsory)
- Salt and pepper, as needed

Instructions:

1. Chicken breasts may be grilled on a grill or in a pan up to done. Slice into thin strips.
2. Combine Romaine lettuce, Parmesan cheese, and Caesar dressing in a big bowl.
3. Divide the salad Mixture among the tortillas after they have been laid out.
4. Add split chicken and, if using, croutons on top. Add salt and pepper for seasoning.
5. Serve the tortillas after rolling them into wraps.

Nutrition (per serving):

Cals: 500 kcal, Protein: 35g

Carbs: 40g, Fat: 25g

Fiber: 5g

41.SPINACH AND FETA STUFFED CHICKEN BREASTS

Ingredients:

- 4 boneless, skinless chicken breasts
- 1 cup of fresh spinach, chop-up
- ½ cup of feta cheese, crumbled
- 1 clove garlic, chop-up
- 2 tbsp olive oil
- Salt and pepper as needed
- 1 tsp dried oregano
- ½ tsp paprika

Instructions:

1. Turn the oven on to 375°F, or 190°C.
2. Combine the spinach, feta, oregano, garlic, salt, and pepper in a bowl.
3. Fill every chicken breast with the spinach and feta Mixture after carefully sliceting a pocket in it.
4. Sprinkle the chicken's exterior with salt, pepper, and paprika.
5. In a Big ovenproof skillet, heat the olive oil over medium-high heat.
6. Sear every chicken breast up to golden brown, 3–4 mins per side.
7. The chicken Must be cooked through after 20 to 25 mins of baking in the oven (internal temperature Must be 165°F/75°C).
8. Serve right away.

Nutrition (per serving):

Cals: 290, Protein: 34g

Fat: 15g, Carbs: 4g

Fiber: 1g, Sugar: 2g

42.CHEAP AND CHEESY BEEF TACOS

Prep Time: 10 mins
Cook Time: 15 mins
Total Time: 25 mins
Servings: 4

Ingredients:

- 1 lb ground beef
- 1 packet taco seasoning (or homemade seasoning combine)
- 2 tbsp water
- 8 mini flour or corn tortillas
- 1 cup of shredded cheddar cheese
- 1 cup of lettuce, shredded
- ½ cup of diced tomatoes
- ¼ cup of sour cream (non-compulsory)
- ¼ cup of salsa (non-compulsory)

Instructions:

1. Using a spoon, break up the ground beef while it browns in a pan over medium heat.
2. Add water and taco seasoning after draining any extra fat. After combineing everything together, simmer for five mins.
3. Use a microwave or dry pan to reheat the tortillas.
4. Spoon the meat Mixture over every tortilla to assemble the tacos.
5. Add salsa, sour cream, tomatoes, lettuce, and cheese on top.
6. Serve right away.

Nutrition (per serving, 2 tacos):

Cals: 350, Protein: 20g, Fat: 20g

Carbs: 25g, Fiber: 3g

Sugar: 4g

43.SIMPLE POTATO AND LEEK SOUP

Prep Time: 10 mins
Cook Time: 30 mins
Total Time: 40 mins
Servings: 4

Ingredients:

- 4 medium potatoes, peel off and diced
- 2 leeks, cleaned and split
- 1 mini onion, diced

- 2 cloves garlic, chop-up
- 4 cups of vegetable or chicken broth
- 2 tbsp butter
- Salt and pepper as needed
- 1 cup of heavy cream (non-compulsory)
- Fresh parsley for garnish (non-compulsory)

Instructions:

1. Melt the butter in a big saucepan over medium heat. Add the garlic, onion, and leeks. Cook up to softened, stirring periodically, for 5 mins.
2. Add the broth and chop-up potatoes. Bring to a boil, then lower the heat and simmer up to the potatoes are soft, about 20 mins.
3. Blend the soup in batches in a blender or with an immersion blender up to it's smooth.
4. Add the cream (if using), simmer for another five mins, and season with salt and pepper.
5. If preferred, top with fresh parsley and serve hot.

Nutrition (per serving):

Cals: 210, Protein: 4g

Fat: 12g, Carbs: 25g

Fiber: 3g, Sugar: 3g

44. MUSHROOM RISOTTO ON A BUDGET

Prep Time: 10 mins
Cook Time: 30 mins
Total Time: 40 mins
Servings: 4

Ingredients:

- 1 cup of Arborio rice
- 2 cups of mushrooms, split
- 1 mini onion, diced
- 2 cloves garlic, chop-up
- 4 cups of vegetable or chicken broth
- ½ cup of finely grated Parmesan cheese
- 2 tbsp olive oil

- Salt and pepper as needed
- 1 tbsp butter (non-compulsory)

Instructions:

1. Heat the olive oil in a big skillet over medium heat. Cook the garlic and onion for three to four mins, or up to they are tender.
2. Cook the mushrooms for five more mins, or up to they are tender.
3. Add the Arborio rice and heat, stirring, up to the rice is gently toasted, about 2 mins.
4. Add the broth gradually, half a cup of at a time, stirring continuously up to the liquid is absorbed, and then add more.
5. Add more liquid and stir up to the rice is creamy and soft, which Must take 20 to 25 mins.
6. Add the butter (if using) and Parmesan cheese, and season with salt and pepper.
7. Serve right away.

Nutrition (per serving):

Cals: 300, Protein: 7g

Fat: 12g, Carbs: 40g

Fiber: 2g, Sugar: 3g

45.CHICKPEA AND SPINACH CURRY

Prep Time: 10 mins
Cook Time: 20 mins
Total Time: 30 mins
Servings: 4

Ingredients:

- 1 can (15 oz) chickpeas, drained and rinsed
- 3 cups of fresh spinach, chop-up
- 1 onion, diced
- 2 cloves garlic, chop-up
- 1 tbsp ginger, finely grated
- 1 tbsp curry powder
- 1 tsp cumin
- 1 can (14 oz) diced tomatoes
- 1 can (14 oz) coconut milk
- 2 tbsp olive oil
- Salt and pepper as needed
- Fresh cilantro for garnish (non-compulsory)

Instructions:

1. In a Big pan, heat the olive oil over medium heat. Cook the ginger, garlic, and onion for three to four mins, or up to they are tender.
2. Cook for one more min after adding the cumin and curry powder.
3. Stir in the coconut milk, tomatoes, and chickpeas. Cook for ten mins after bringing to a simmer.
4. Cook the spinach for about two mins, or up to it has wilted.
5. If preferred, top with fresh cilantro and season with salt and pepper to suit.
6. Serve over naan or rice.

Nutrition (per serving):

Cals: 350, Protein: 12g

Fat: 18g, Carbs: 42g

Fiber: 10g, Sugar: 8g

Prep Time: 15 mins

Cook Time: 10 mins

Total Time: 25 mins

Servings: 4

Ingredients:

- 1 tbsp olive oil
- 1 onion, diced
- 1 bell pepper, diced
- 1 zucchini, diced
- 1 cup of corn kernels (fresh or refrigerate)
- 1 can black beans, drained and rinsed
- 1 tsp chili powder
- 1 tsp cumin
- Salt and pepper as needed
- 8 mini flour tortillas
- 1/2 cup of shredded lettuce
- 1/2 cup of diced tomatoes
- 1/4 cup of fresh cilantro, chop-up
- 1/4 cup of sour cream (non-compulsory)
- Lime wedges for serving

Instructions:

1. In a Big skillet, heat the olive oil over medium heat.
2. Add the bell pepper, zucchini, and onion. Cook for approximately five mins, or up to tender.
3. Add cumin, chili powder, black beans, corn, salt, and pepper. Cook for a further five mins, stirring, up to well cooked.
4. Use a microwave or a dry skillet to reheat tortillas.
5. Put the tacos together: Top with lettuce, tomatoes, cilantro, and sour cream after spooning the vegetable Mixture onto the tortillas.
6. Serve with slices of lime.

Nutrition (per serving):

Cals: 300, Protein: 10g

Carbs: 48g, Fat: 9g

Fiber: 8g

47. BUDGET-FRIENDLY BEEF AND BEAN BURRITOS

Prep Time: 10 mins

Cook Time: 20 mins

Total Time: 30 mins

Servings: 4

Ingredients:

- 1 lb ground beef
- 1 tbsp olive oil
- 1 onion, diced
- 2 cloves garlic, chop-up
- 1 can black beans, drained and rinsed
- 1 can diced tomatoes with green chilies
- 1 tsp chili powder
- 1 tsp cumin
- Salt and pepper as needed
- 4 Big flour tortillas
- 1 cup of shredded cheddar cheese
- 1/2 cup of sour cream (non-compulsory)

Instructions:

1. In a Big skillet, heat the olive oil over medium heat. Using a spoon, break up the ground meat while it cooks up to browned.
2. Add the chop-up garlic and onion to the skillet. Cook up to tender, 3–4 mins.
3. Add chop-up tomatoes, cumin, chili powder, black beans, salt, and pepper and stir. Cook for five more mins.
4. Use a microwave or a dry skillet to reheat tortillas.
5. Put the burritos together: Top every tortilla with a spoonful of the meat and bean Mixture. Add sour cream and cheese on top.
6. Serve the burritos after rolling them up.

Nutrition (per serving):

Cals: 450, Protein: 30g

Carbs: 45g, Fat: 20g

Fiber: 8g

48. GROUND TURKEY TACOS

Prep Time: 10 mins

Cook Time: 15 mins

Total Time: 25 mins

Servings: 4

Ingredients:

- 1 lb ground turkey
- 1 tbsp olive oil
- 1 onion, diced
- 1 bell pepper, diced
- 1 tbsp taco seasoning
- 1/2 cup of water
- 8 mini corn or flour tortillas
- 1/2 cup of shredded lettuce
- 1/2 cup of diced tomatoes
- 1/4 cup of shredded cheddar cheese
- 1/4 cup of salsa

Instructions:

1. In a pan, heat the olive oil over medium heat. Add the ground turkey and sauté up to browned, breaking it up with a spoon.
2. Add the bell pepper and split onion. Cook for approximately five mins, or up to tender.
3. Add the water and taco seasoning and stir. Simmer up to the Mixture thickens, about 5 mins.
4. Use a microwave or a dry skillet to reheat tortillas.
5. Put the tacos together: Place a spoonful of the turkey Mixture on every tortilla. Add salsa, cheese, tomatoes, and lettuce on top.
6. Serve right away.

Nutrition (per serving):

Cals: 350, Protein: 30g

Carbs: 30g, Fat: 15g

Fiber: 5g

Made in the USA
Middletown, DE
23 May 2025

75972708R00031